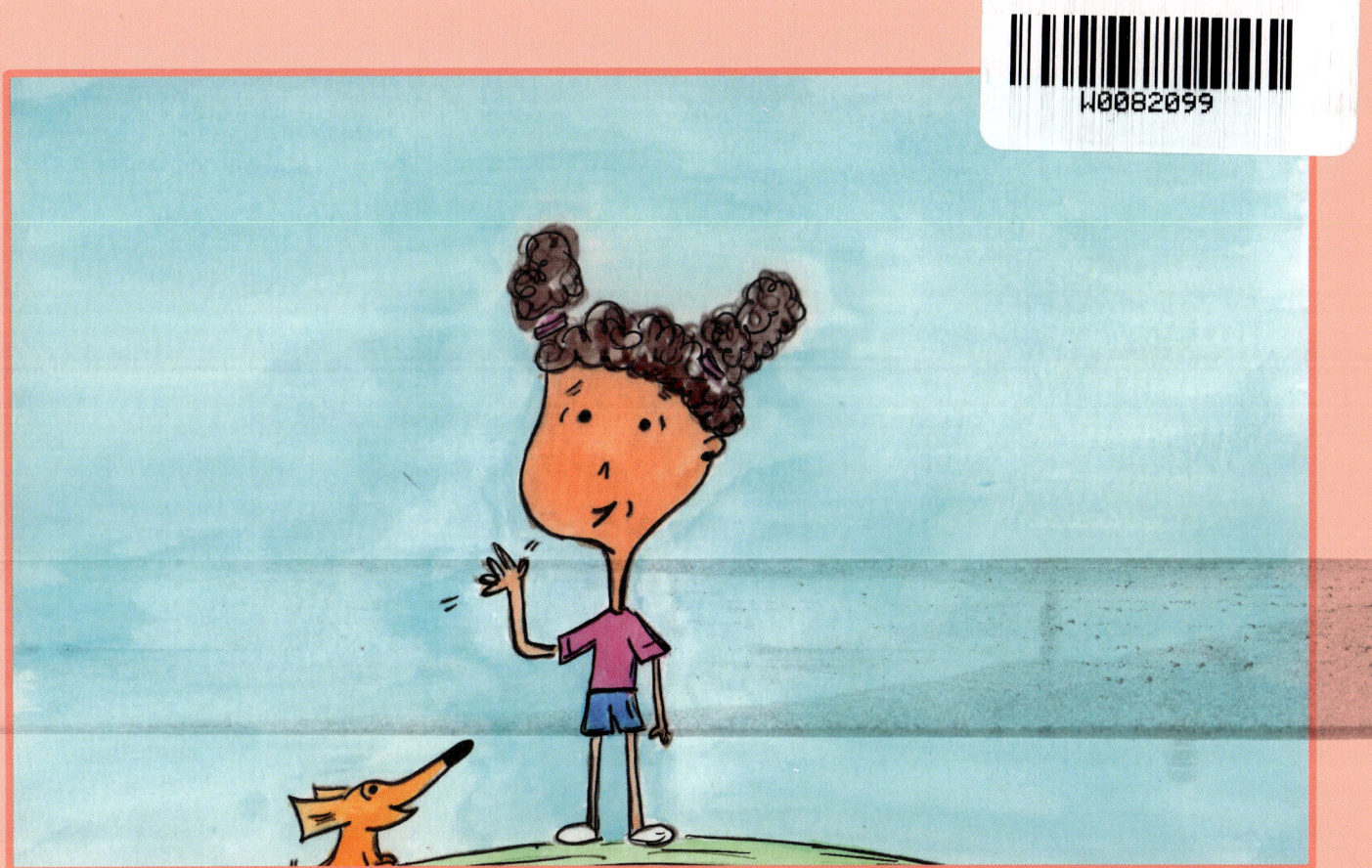

Hi there! My name is Tiana, and I am here to tell you all about **peritoneal dialysis**. Because maybe you need dialysis...or maybe you know someone who does.

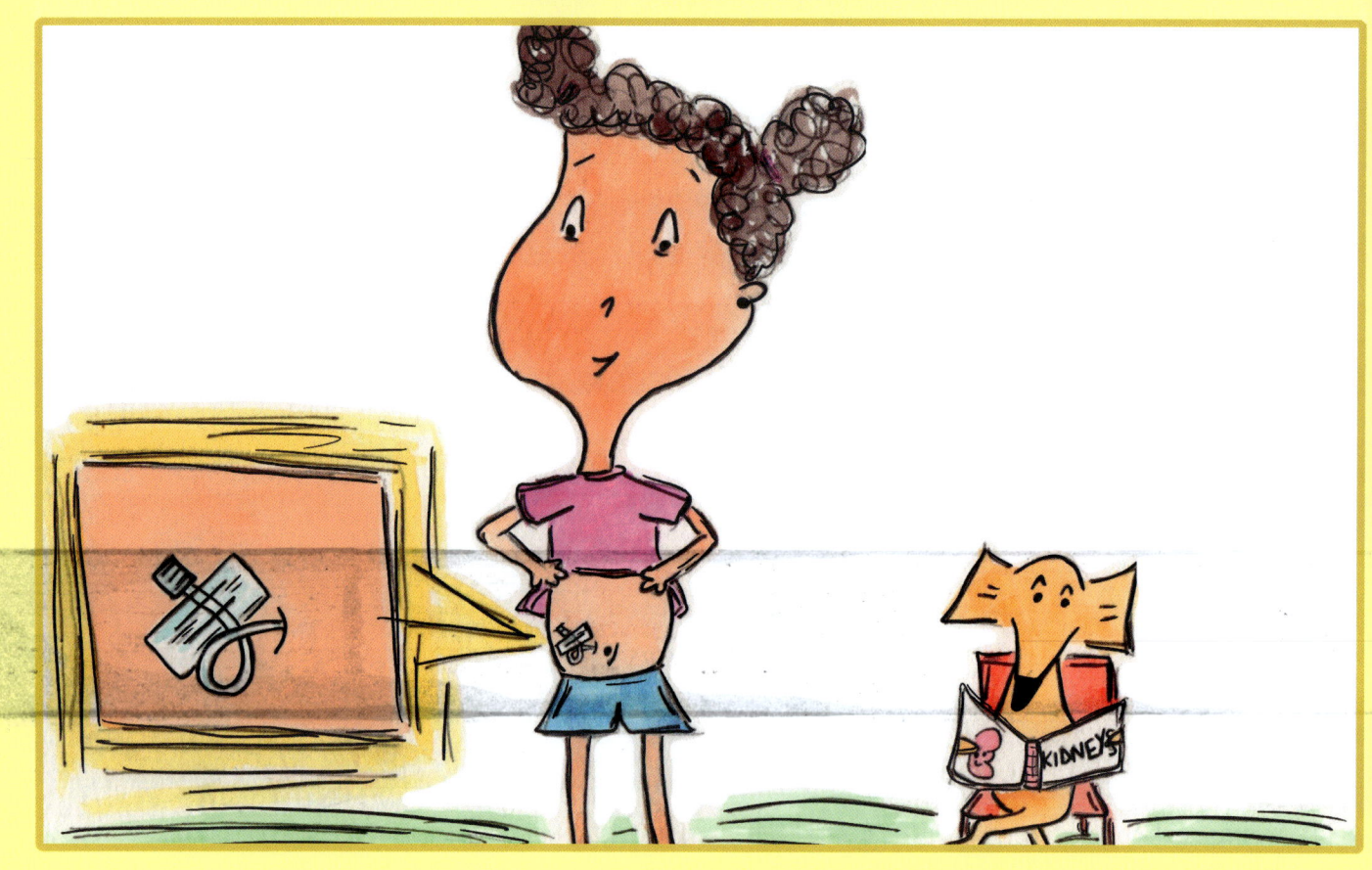

Pear-it-toe-neal Di – al – uh – sis. First off, what is it?
It is a special treatment for people, like me, who need help
cleaning their blood. Now wait a second.
Why does our blood need to be cleaned?
Great question! To answer that,
we have to talk about kidneys.

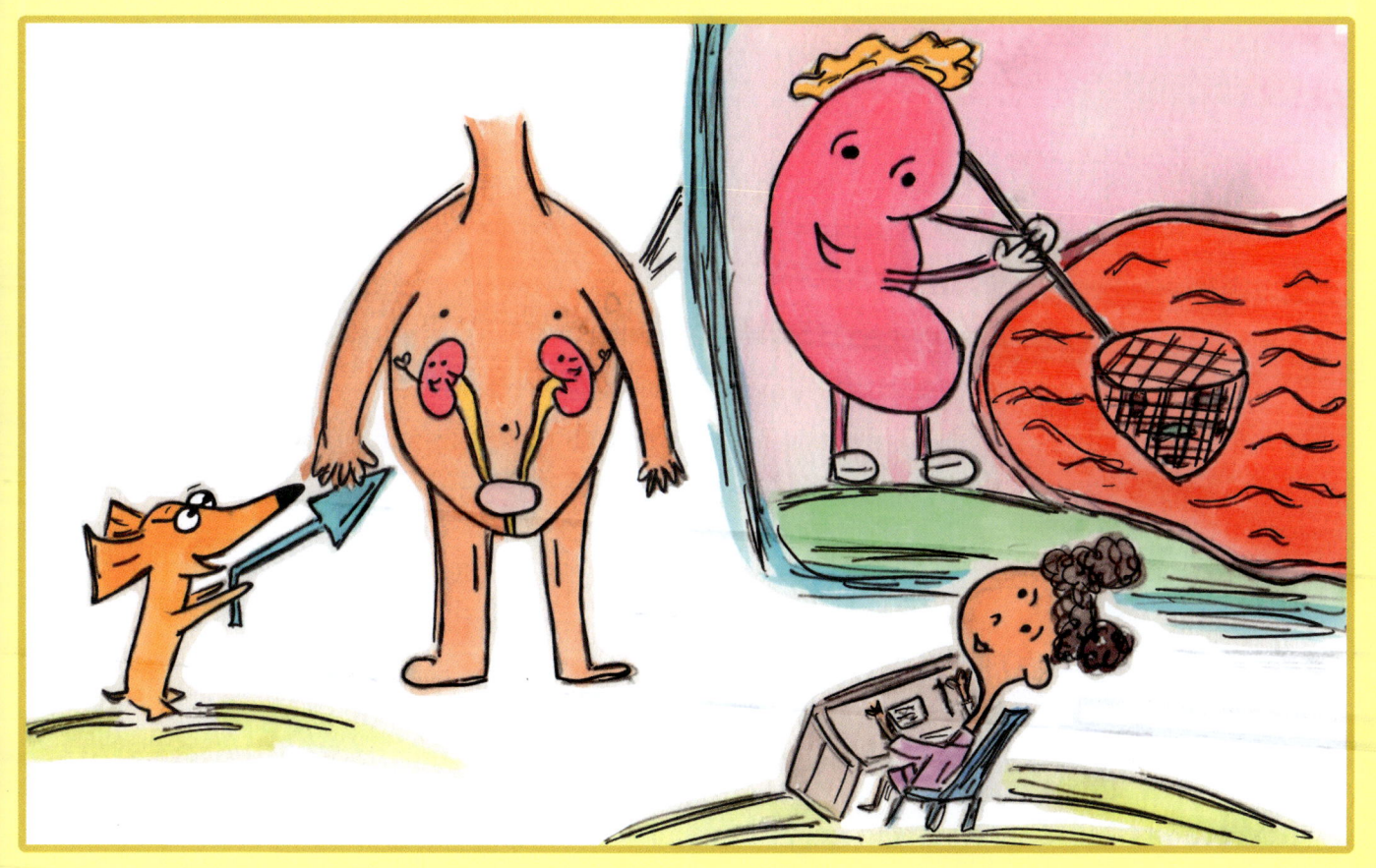

Kidneys are organs in our bodies. Most people are born with two! They look like kidney beans and their main job is to clean our blood and help remove waste, extra salt, and water from the body. When we eat and drink, our bodies break down our foods and liquids into different parts.

Some of these parts are like trash – full of dirty stuff that our bodies do not need and must get rid of.

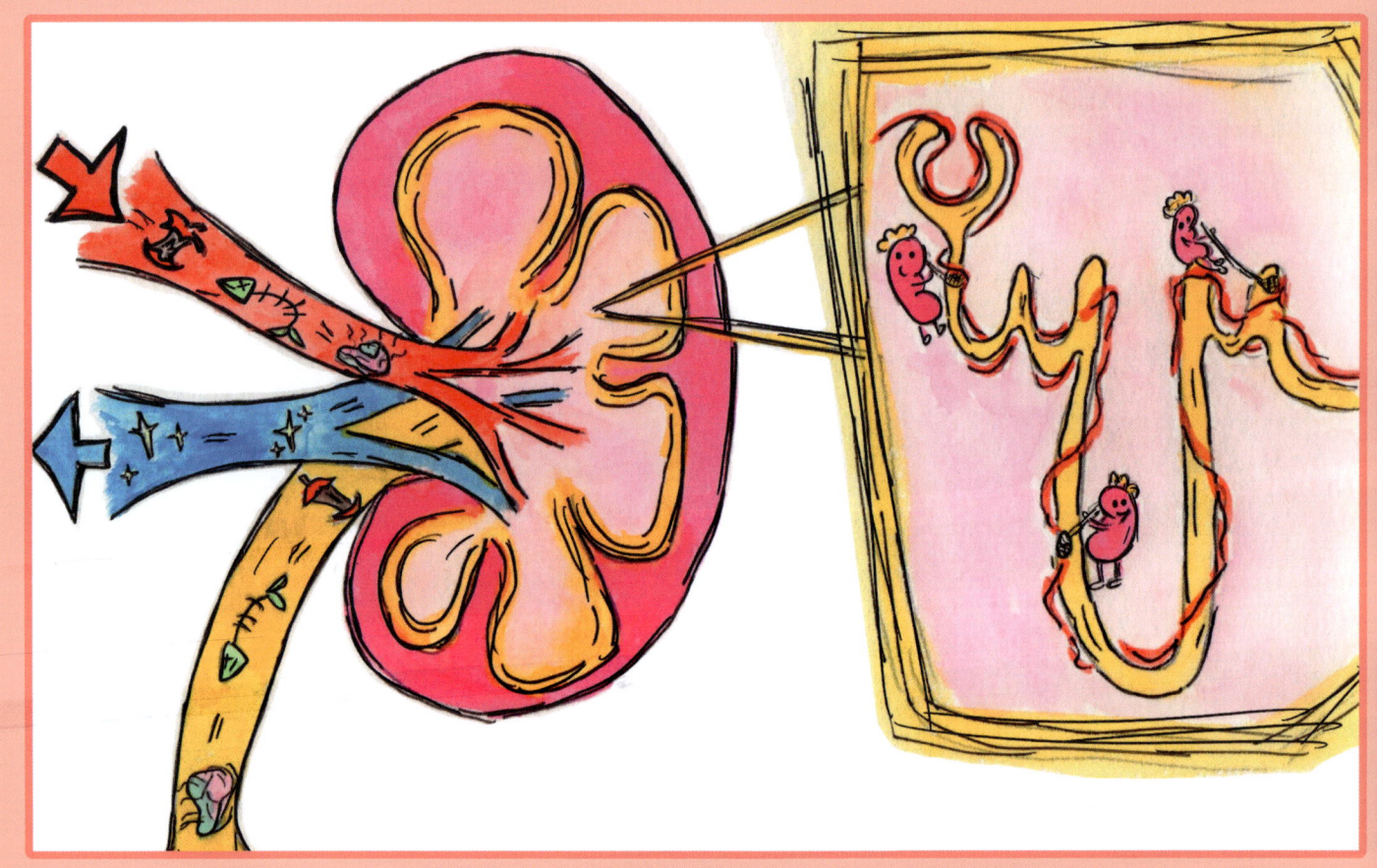

The "trash" travels in our blood to our kidneys. As it passes through our kidneys, the dirty stuff is pulled out and becomes part of our **urine** (also known as 'pee').
This is how our blood is cleaned! We then pee out all that dirty stuff from our blood. Our blood is now clean and can continue to help our bodies.

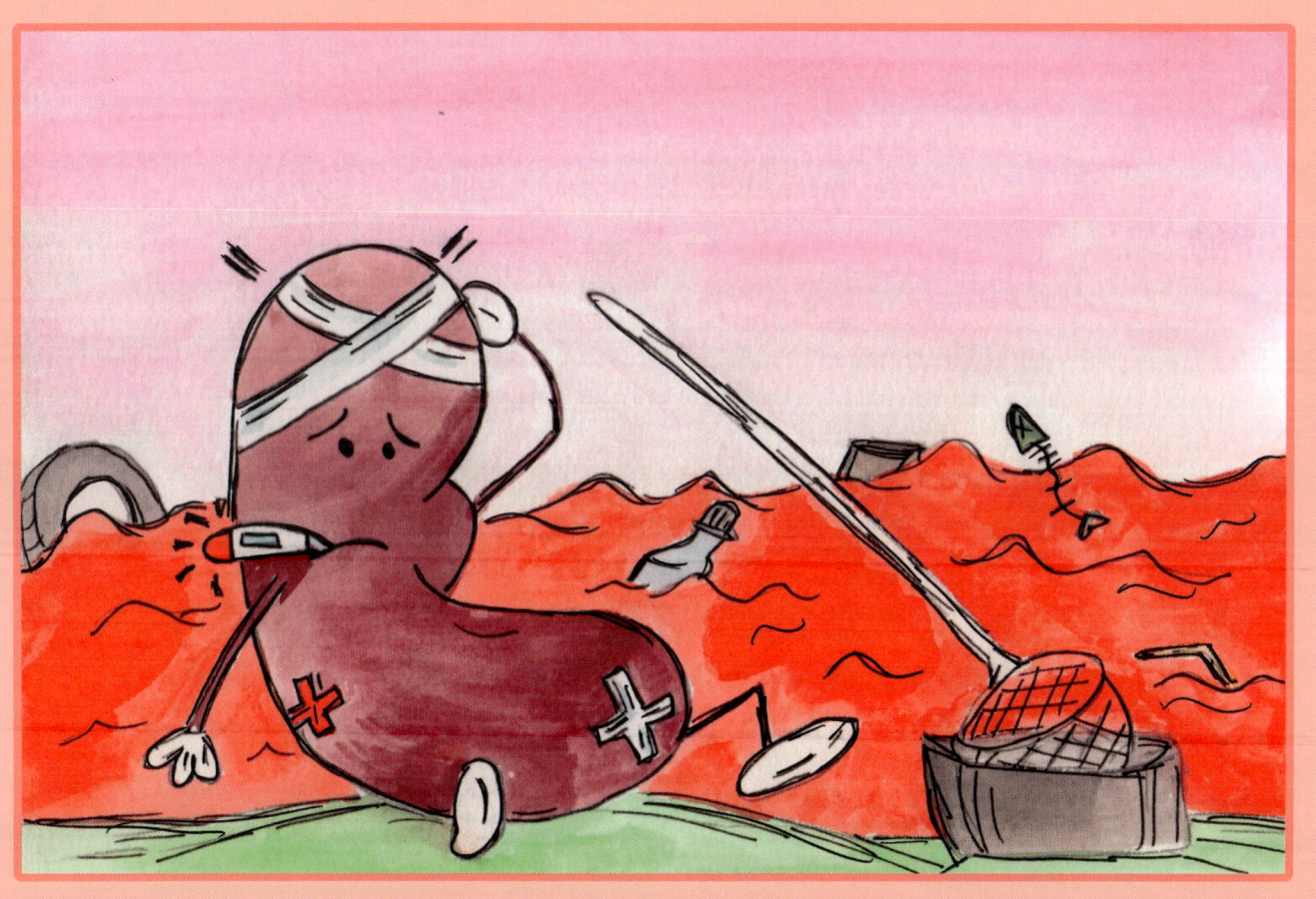

Now some of us have kidneys that do not work as well, so
sometimes they have trouble cleaning our blood.
So, our blood gets dirtier and dirtier.
And dirty blood makes us feel sick.
How can we help our kidneys clean our blood
and feel better?

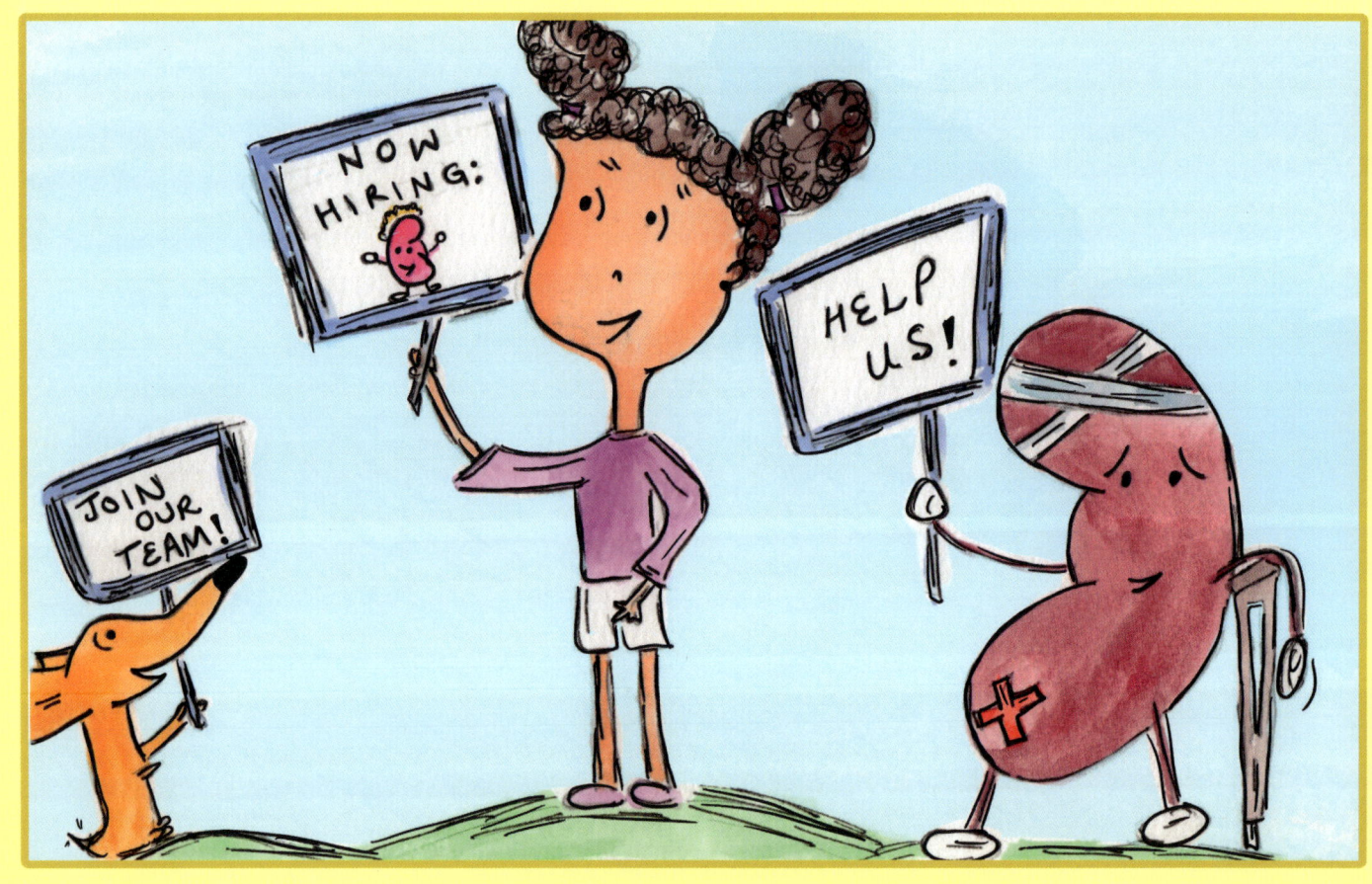

What we really need is a new kidney. But getting a new kidney can take time. Until then, we can use **peritoneal dialysis**. What is it?
I like to think of peritoneal dialysis as a bath for our bellies. Let me explain.

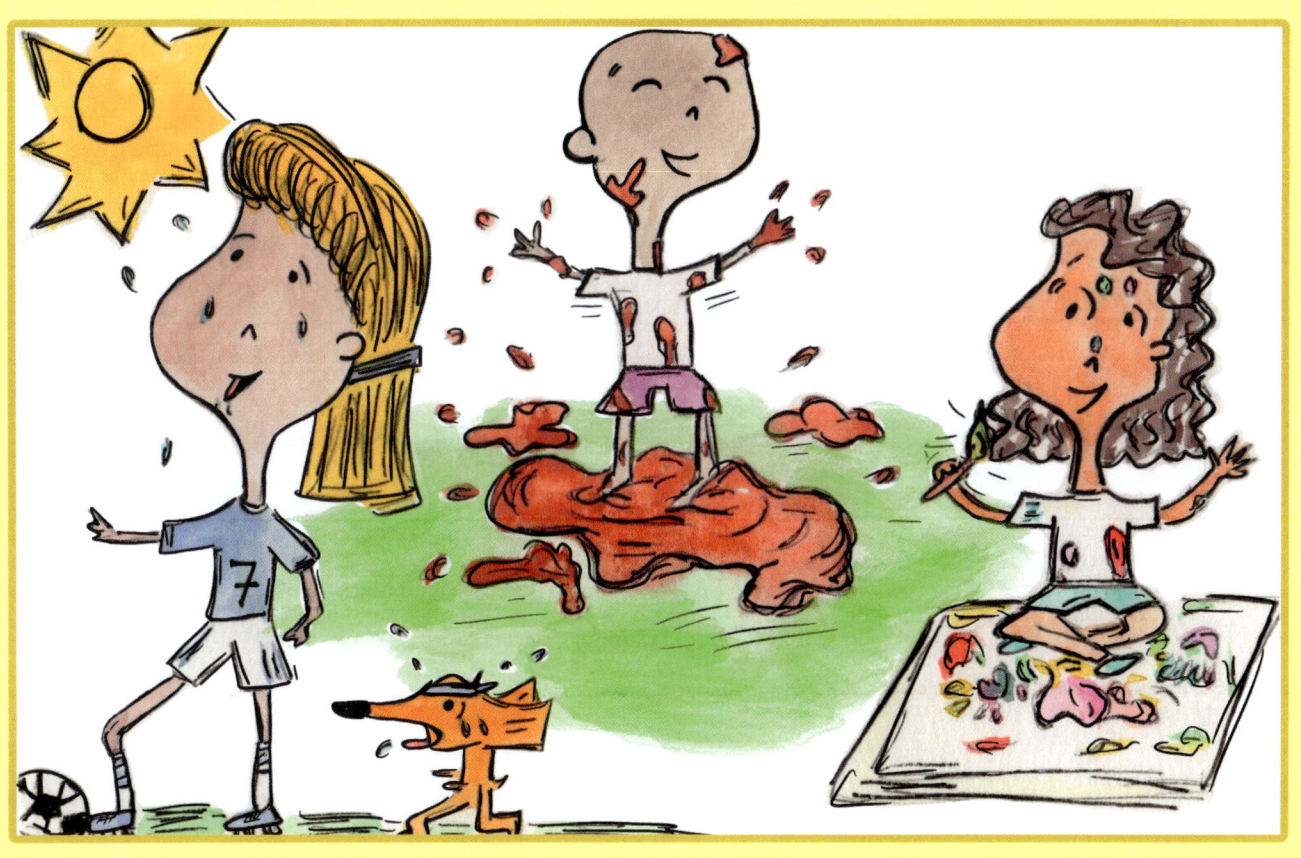

When we play outside on a hot day, we might get sweaty and dirty. We might also play in sticky mud, eat a messy meal, or paint a splashy painting, making us extra dirty!

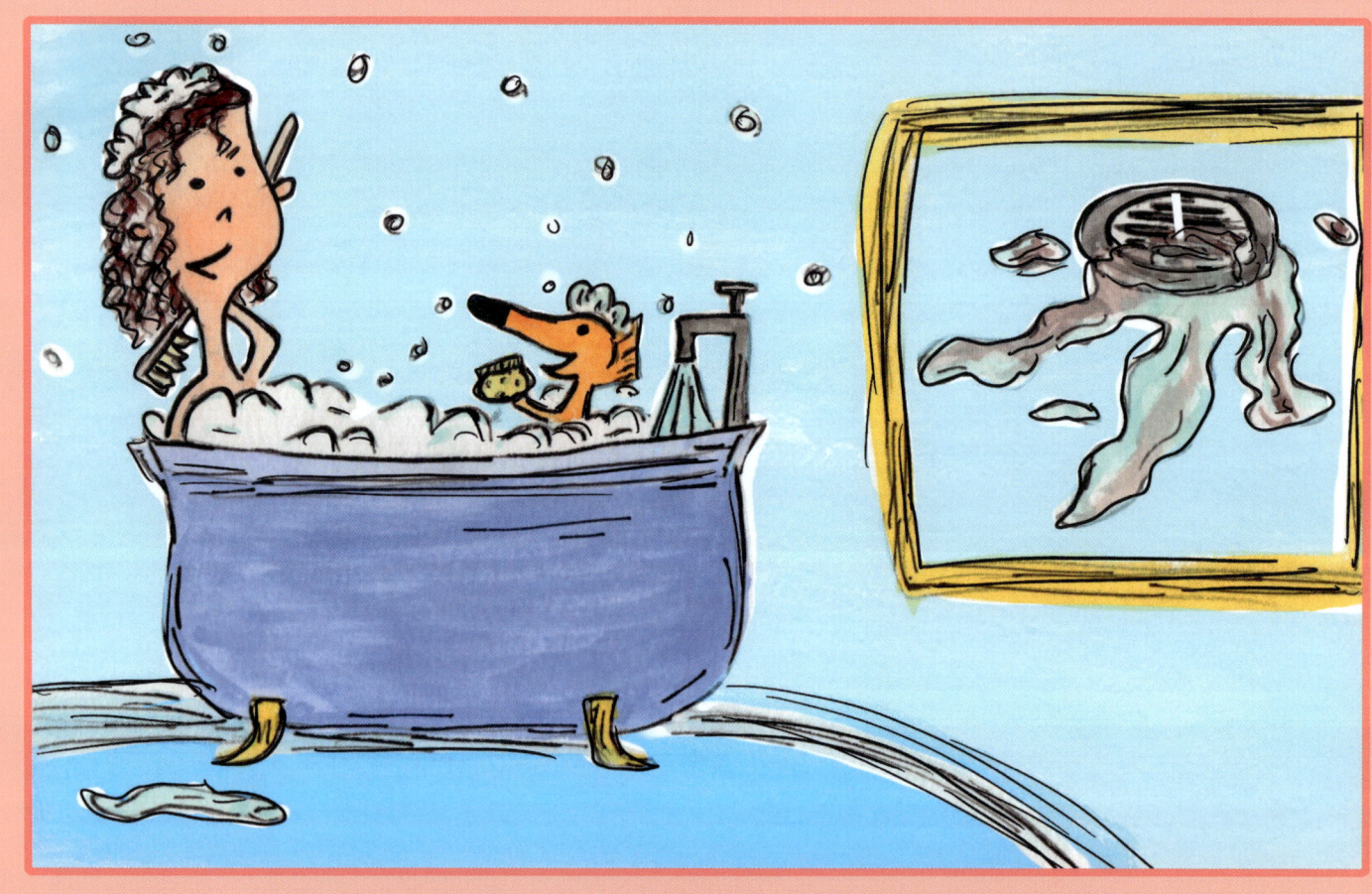

This calls for a bath to clean up our bodies.

I like to soak in the clean, soapy, warm water.

Let it splish splash all over me, washing away the dirt and sweat.

And then the dirty water swirls down the drain, leaving me fresh and clean!

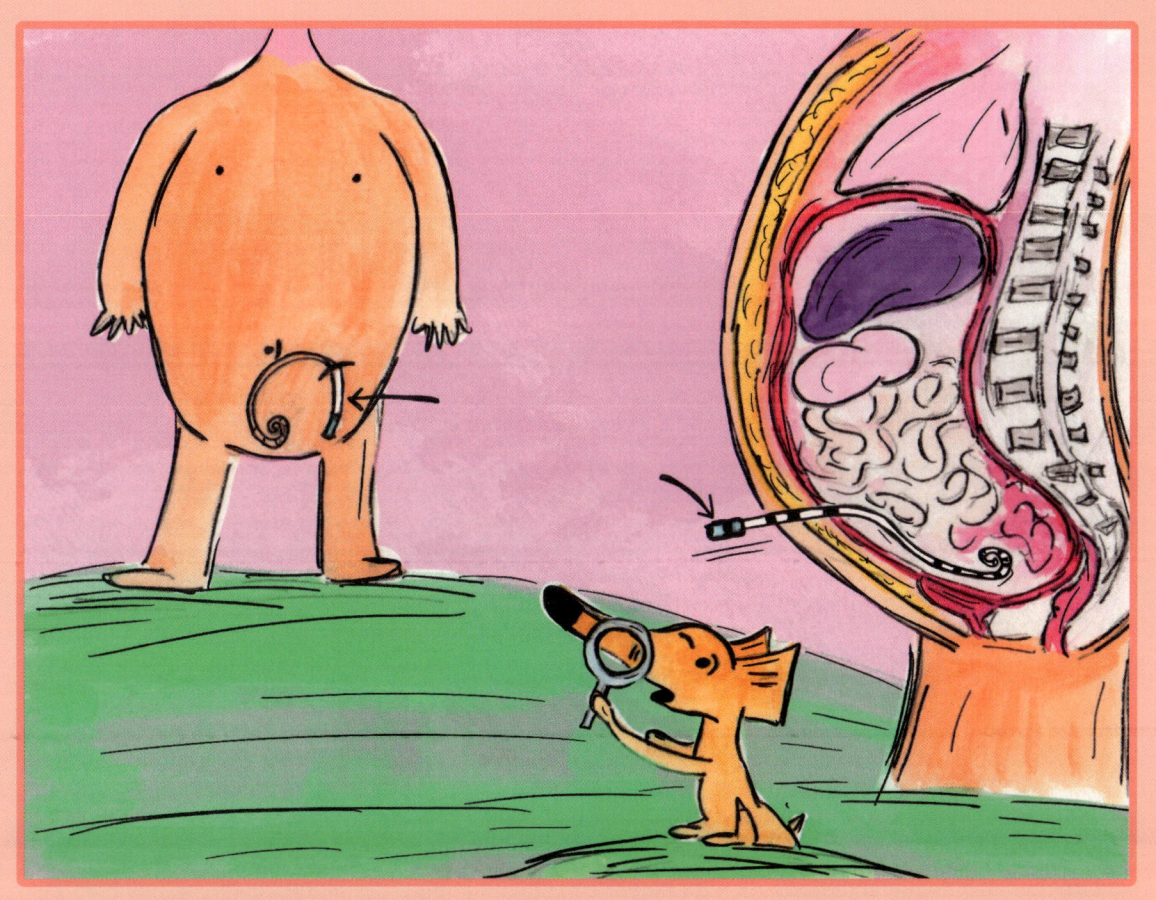

Peritoneal dialysis does the same thing as a bath!
It cleans our blood just like a bath cleans our bodies.
First, a tube is placed into your belly by a surgeon.
You will be sound asleep and will not feel a thing.
When you wake up, it will hurt a little at first.

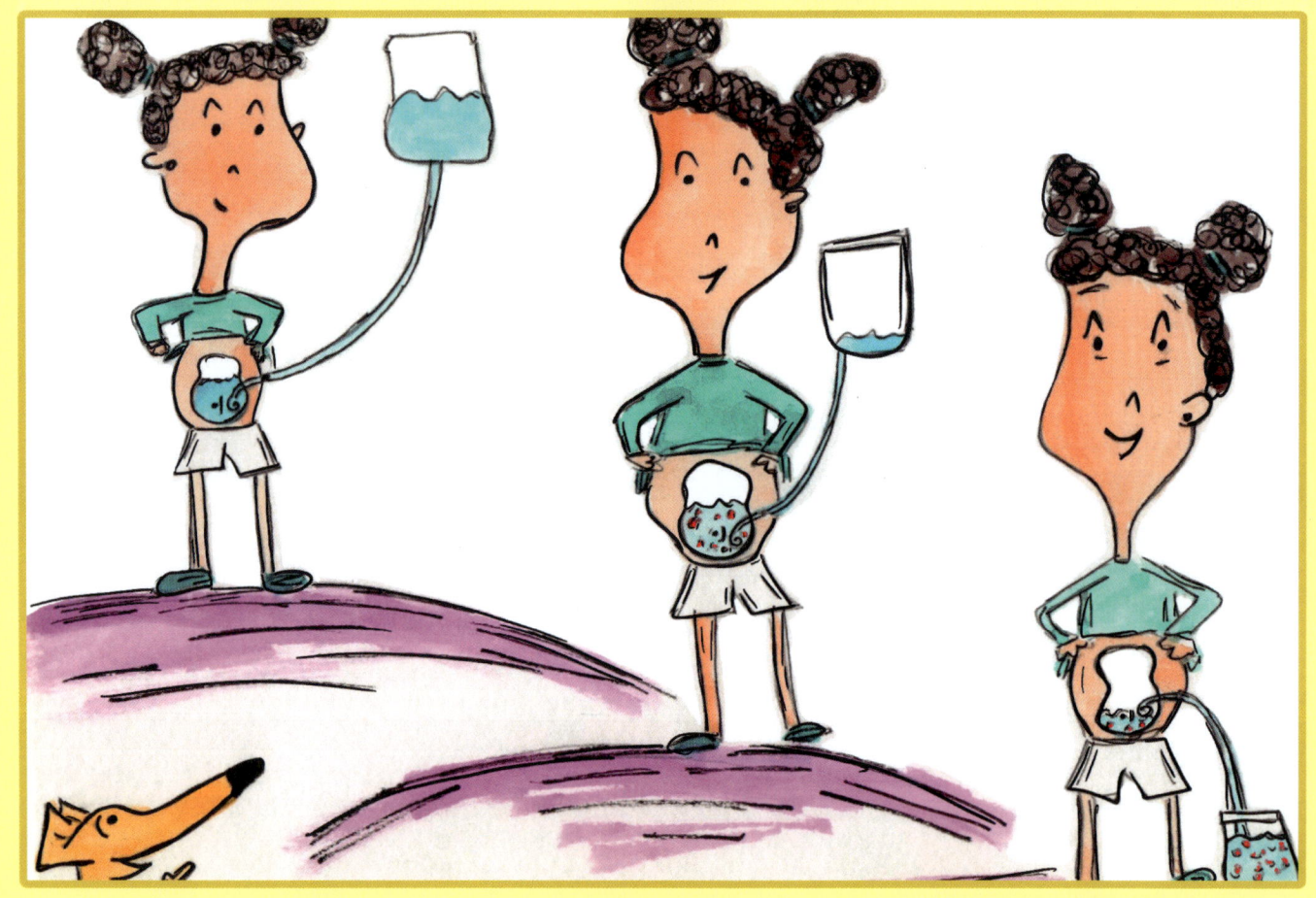

After two weeks, it's time to use the tube! A special cleaning liquid called **dialysate** is put into the tube, and travels into your belly. It then swishes around your belly, collecting all the dirty stuff from your blood. It doesn't hurt, but your belly may feel a little full while this happens.

Then the liquid drains back out, leaving your body. Bye-bye!

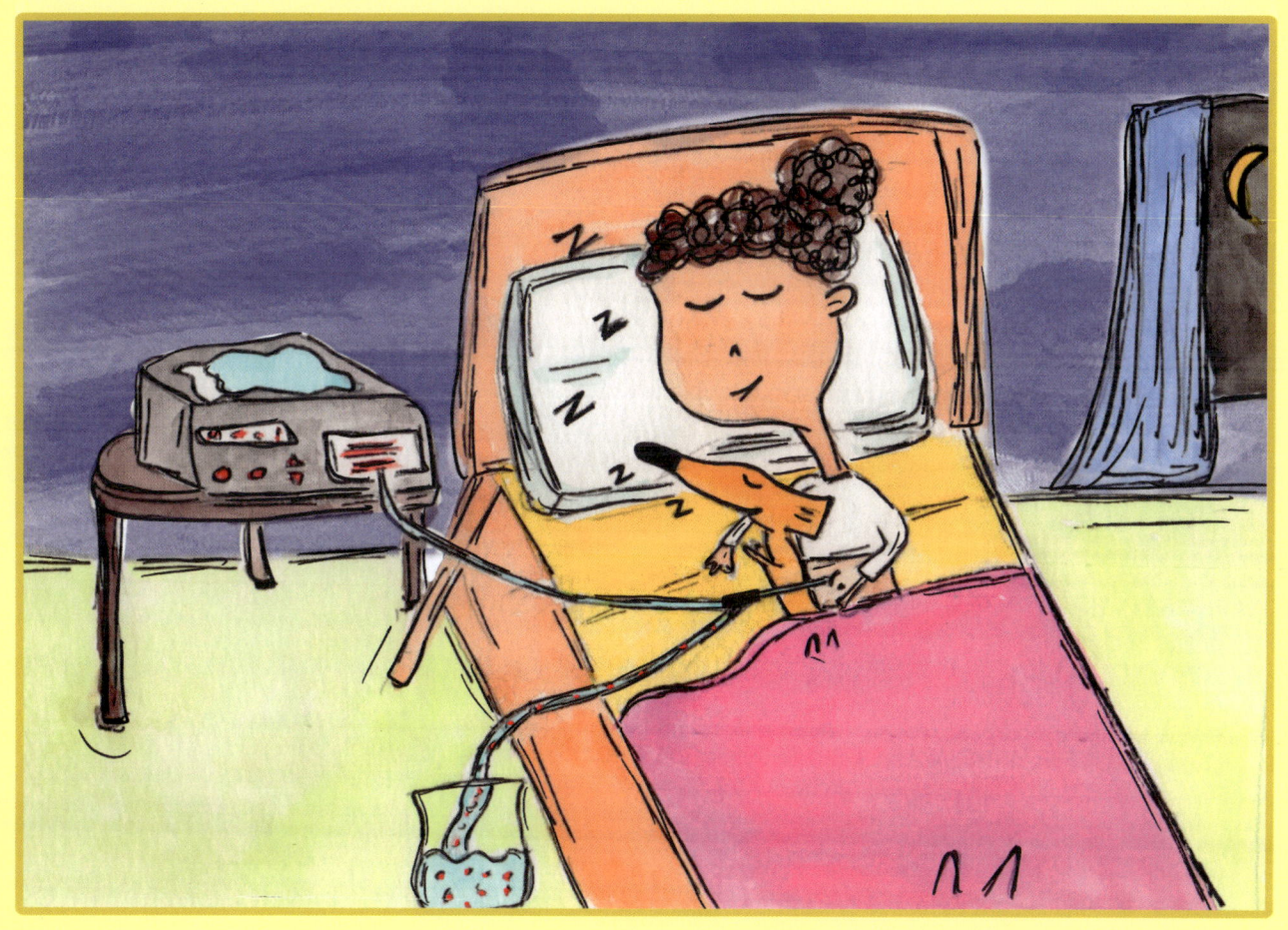

You can clean your blood with peritoneal dialysis at any time, and at any place. You can do it in the car, in the airport, in the park, or even at an amusement park! While you're doing it, you can read, watch a movie, or even play video games! I like to do it at home while I sleep. So, when I wake up, it's all done, and my blood is clean!

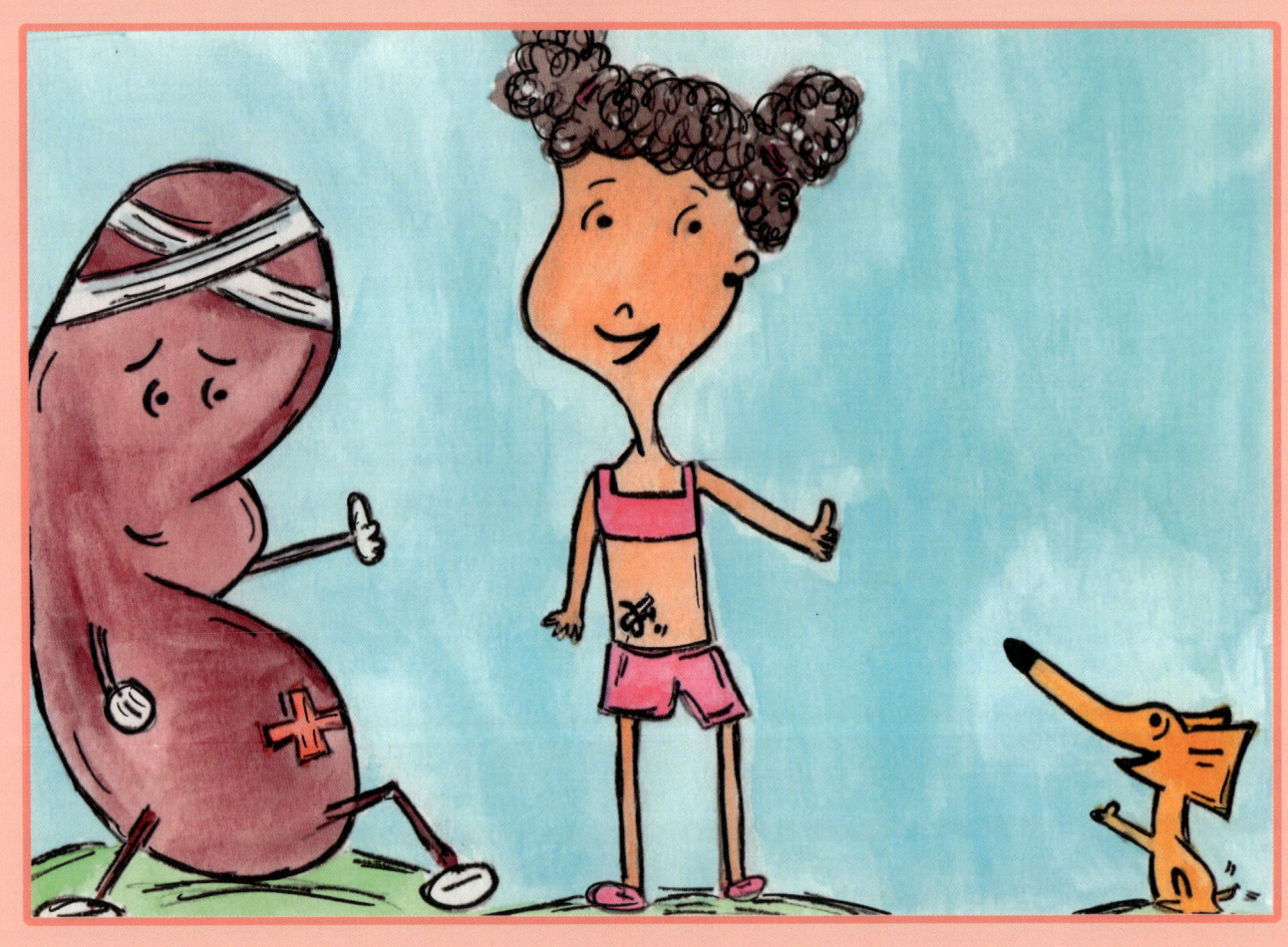

So you see, peritoneal dialysis helps people like me, and many others, who have kidneys that don't work as well.
It helps us stay healthy, and clean,
until a new kidney is found.
A bath for our bellies!

Kidney & Dialysis Facts

Our kidneys keep our blood clean by removing extra water, salt, and chemicals. They clean our blood multiple times – every hour!

Our kidneys are also in charge of making **Vitamin D** (which makes your bones strong!), **red blood cell** formation (to prevent anemia-a low blood count), and keeping your **blood pressure** in a good range!

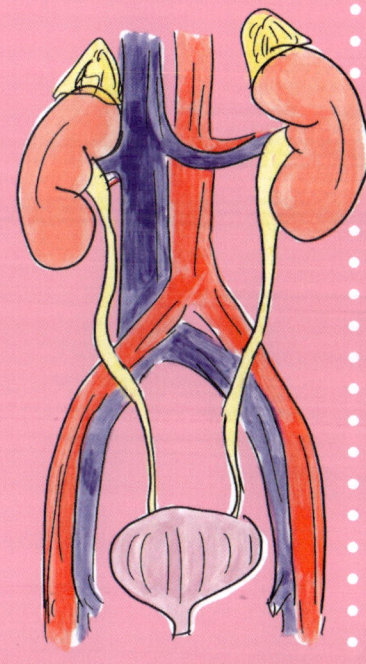

They are hard workers! Kidneys remove the extra water, salt, and chemicals through our pee (**urine**), so that they exit our bodies.

Now what if our kidneys are not working well? The extra water, salt, and chemicals will build up in our blood, instead of exiting through our pee. This is the '**dirty stuff**' that can hurt our bodies and make us feel sick. Some of us are still able to pee. Some of us are not able to pee.

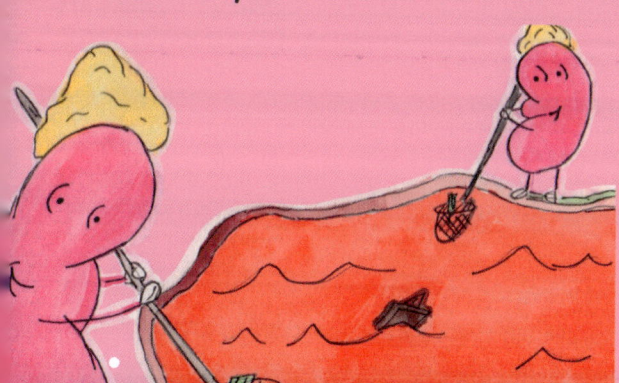

You usually don't feel sick until your kidneys only work **less than 30%** (out of 100%). Even then medicines can help before dialysis is needed.

Feeling sick may include feeling tired, having trouble in school, and not growing. You may have puffiness, electrolyte issues, weak bones, low blood counts (**anemia**), and high blood pressure.

That's where dialysis comes in! **Dialysis** cleans our blood when our kidneys are not able to. Dialysis is not perfect. It can only do part of the kidney's job. But this will help keep our bodies working until a new kidney is found for us (a **kidney transplant**).

There are two types of dialysis:

a) **Hemodialysis** – A machine removes your blood, cleans it by filtering out the 'dirty stuff,' and then returns it back to your body. Usually this takes about 4 hours and is done 3 times a week. Read our book **Dialysis: An Aquarium Filter for your Blood** to learn more!

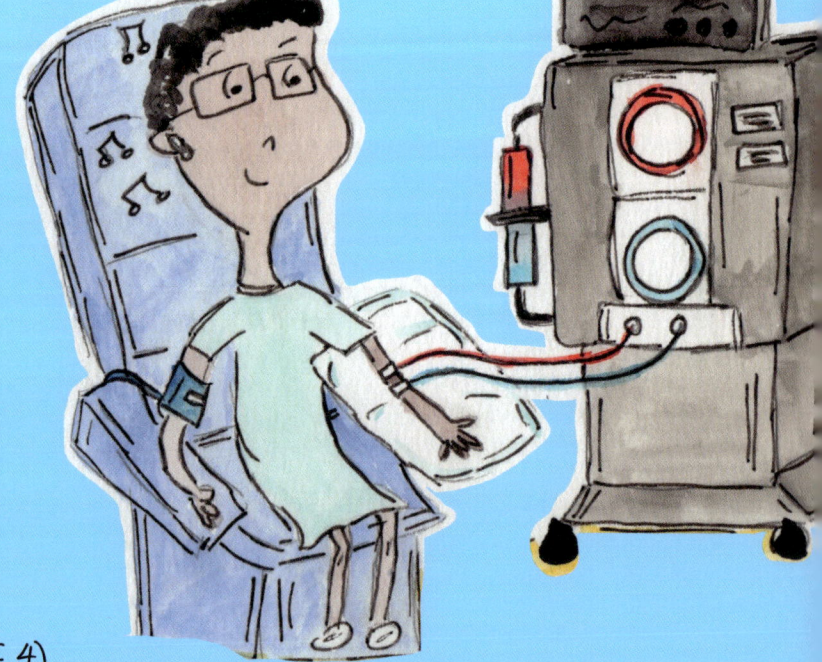

b) **Peritoneal dialysis** — that's what this book is about!

Did you know most kids (3 out of 4) need dialysis before they get a kidney transplant?

The details!

1) **Peritoneal Diaylsis requires a PD catheter.** This is a soft tube that is placed into your belly by a surgeon. It is about as long as a ruler. Part of it sits inside your belly and part of it sits outside your belly.

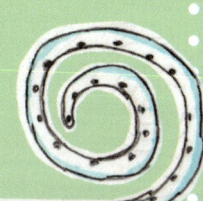

2) **The steps**

   a. Special clear fluid called **dialysate** is put into your belly, through your tube, and sits there for a few hours.

   b. All the 'dirty stuff' from your blood flows through your **peritoneal lining** (the lining of your belly) and into the dialysate fluid.

   c. The fluid sucks in all the 'dirty stuff.'

   d. The now dirty fluid drains back out of the tube, leaving your body (the fluid will still look clear).

3) It can be done **at home** and usually takes 8-10 hours. You can do it at night, while you sleep, or several times a day instead. Make sure to remind your family to write down how much dirty fluid is drained out of your belly.

4) **Diet** is important in peritoneal dialysis. You may need to be on a special diet called a **'renal diet.'** This means you cannot eat certain foods, such as very salty foods. You also may not be able to drink as much as you used to. So, it is important to pay attention to what you eat, and keep track of how much you drink! Ask your doctor for more information!

15

Surgery Facts

A surgeon will put your PD catheter in your belly.

Don't eat anything after midnight the night before your procedure! You can drink water up to 2 hours before.

Placing the catheter takes about 30 minutes.

You will be asleep during it, so you won't feel a thing.

Your surgeon will make a small cut near your belly button and push the tube into your belly. Another small cut is made for the tube's exit site. The tube is pulled from the first cut, under your skin, until it comes out the exit site. This **tunneling** helps keep it in place.

Afterwards, you will have some blue glue over your incision or a bandage. This glue will peel off in several weeks. It helps your cut heal, so do not peel it off on your own.

There will be a special bandage over your PD catheter. Keep it dry and don't remove it. A nurse will remove it after 7-10 days.

You can shower or take a bath after you see the nurse.

You can start your dialysis two weeks after surgery.

Your surgery may not be exactly as described here – each hospital can be a little different!

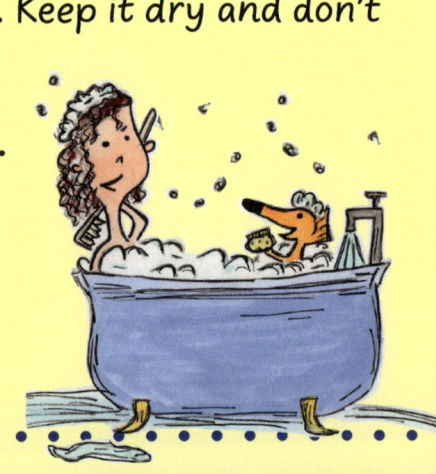

Catheter Care

Your PD catheter needs protection from germs!

Always wash your hands before touching your PD catheter. Scrub them AND sanitize them.

Clean your exit site daily.

Try to avoid wearing tight clothing.

Try to avoid sleeping on your belly.

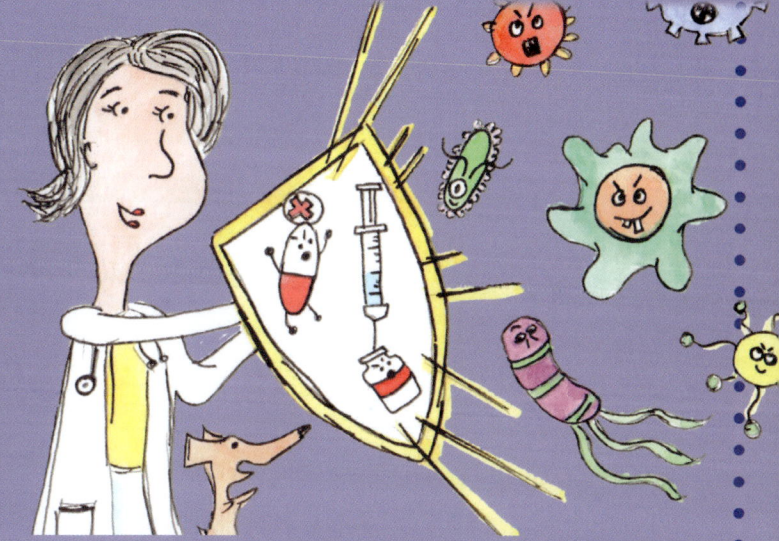

Keep your tube taped down to your belly to keep it from getting pulled on.

Talk to your doctor before swimming in open water (ocean, lakes) or pools. Your doctor will let you know if you should avoid these activities or if you can safely swim by covering your catheter.

Showers and baths are fine!

Call your doctor if there is redness or pain at your tube site.

When your tube is open, everyone should wear a mask to be extra safe. If you have a pet, they should stay in another room until your tube is closed again.

Doctor Words

Kidneys – organs that clean your blood by removing extra water, salt, and chemicals that can hurt you, through your pee. They are also in charge of Vitamin D metabolism (which keeps your bones strong!), red blood cell production (prevents 'anemia', or low blood counts), and keeping your blood pressure in a good range. If your kidneys do not work as well, that's when you need dialysis.

Peritoneum – the lining of your belly (drawn in dark pink). It's like a pillow cover if your belly was a pillow. It filters out 'dirty stuff' from blood.

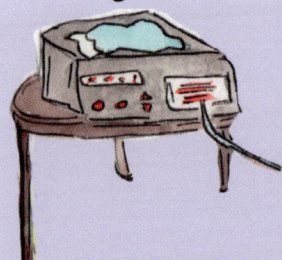

Continuous cyclic peritoneal dialysis (CCPD) – an automatic machine that lets you do your peritoneal dialysis while you are asleep.

Dialysate – the special clean fluid that you put into your body to wash out the 'dirty stuff.'

Hemodialysis — a machine removes your blood, cleans it by filtering out the 'dirty stuff,' and then returns it back to your body.

Acute kidney failure — a previously healthy kidney that gets sick suddenly from illness, medicines, accidents, or poisons. Dialysis may be used for a short period of time to help until your kidney gets better!

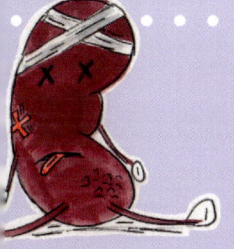

Chronic kidney disease — a kidney problem that gets worse over time. It may eventually lead to end-stage kidney disease.

End-stage kidney disease (ESKD) – when your kidneys don't work as well and are unable to clean your blood; you will need dialysis until you get a kidney transplant. This is also known as 'end stage renal disease' or 'renal failure.'

Deceased donation kidney transplant — when you get a healthy kidney from someone who was really sick or in an accident and died. They no longer need their kidneys. Finding a new kidney through deceased donation can take some time. That's why dialysis is important until then.

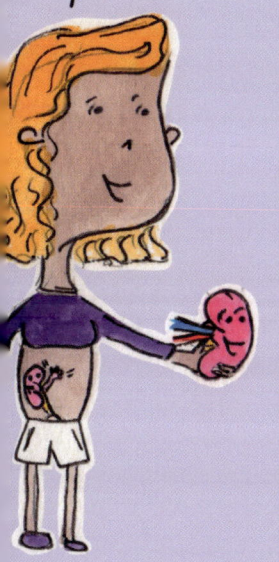

Living donor kidney transplant — this is when a healthy person, like a friend or family member, or even a complete stranger (!) gifts one of their kidneys to you.

Nephrologist — a kidney doctor! They are in charge of taking care of your kidneys when they are sick or after a transplant.

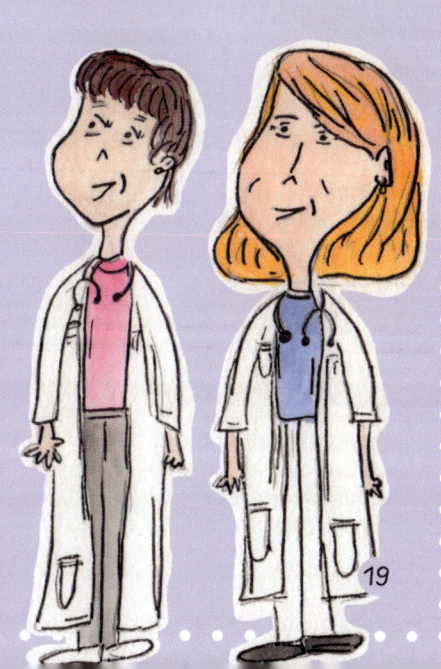

Meet the Author:
Dr. Maria Baimas-George

Maria Baimas-George MD MPH is an abdominal transplant surgeon. Inspired by her patients and mentors, she writes and illustrates books explaining medical and surgical conditions to children and their loved ones. Her goal is to create books that provide useful information to help with understanding and to offer comfort and hope.

WINNER OF THE 2021 SILVER TOUCHSTONE AWARD

Awarded for exceptional performance in patient safety, clinical outcomes, efficiency & service excellence

Please visit us online at
www.StrengthOfMyScars.com to learn more about our team and story and see our full collection of available books.

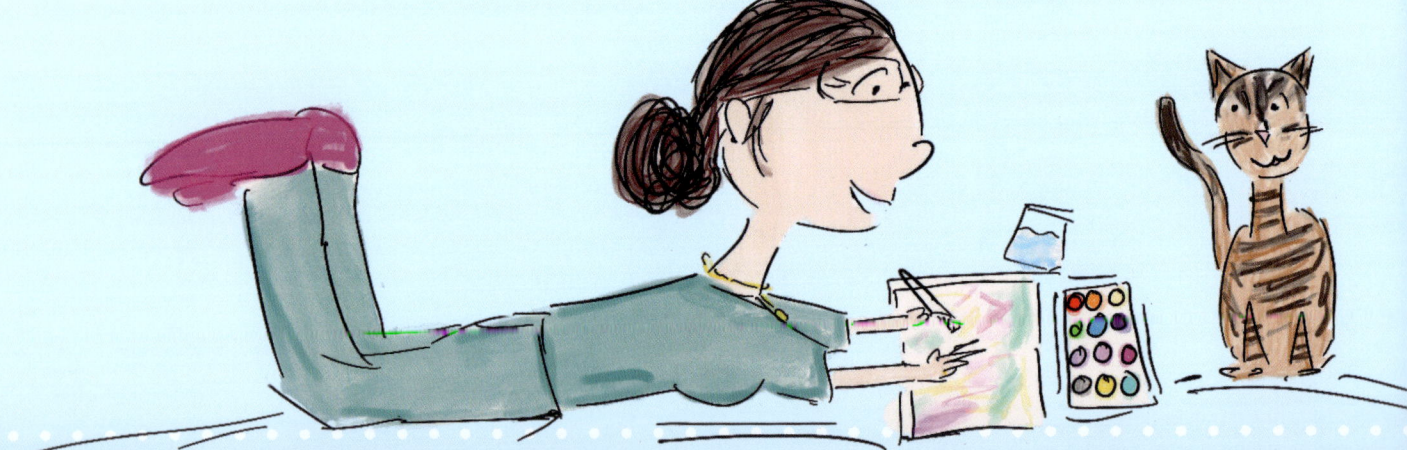

Edited by Lianna Baimas-George

This book was originally created with the support of **Heidi Yeh, MD** and **Susan Massengill, MD.**

Dr. Yeh is not only the **Surgical Director of Pediatric Transplant** at Mass General for Children but has also become an incredible mentor and advocate for Dr. Baimas-George's work in both transplant and writing books.

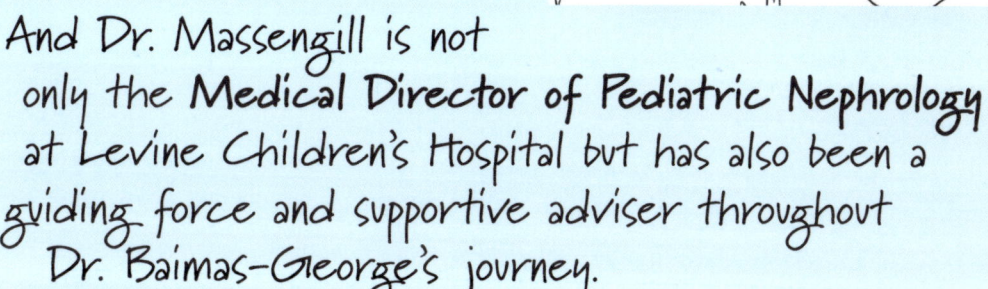

And Dr. Massengill is not only the **Medical Director of Pediatric Nephrology** at Levine Children's Hospital but has also been a guiding force and supportive adviser throughout Dr. Baimas-George's journey.

Both were instrumental for their subject-matter expert review & edits of this book.

We would also like to thank **Barb Luby** LICSW of Mass General for Children Transplant Center for her support and edits and **Brianna Cimino** and **Martin Dafov**, our patient reviewers, for using their experience with peritoneal dialysis to improve this book.

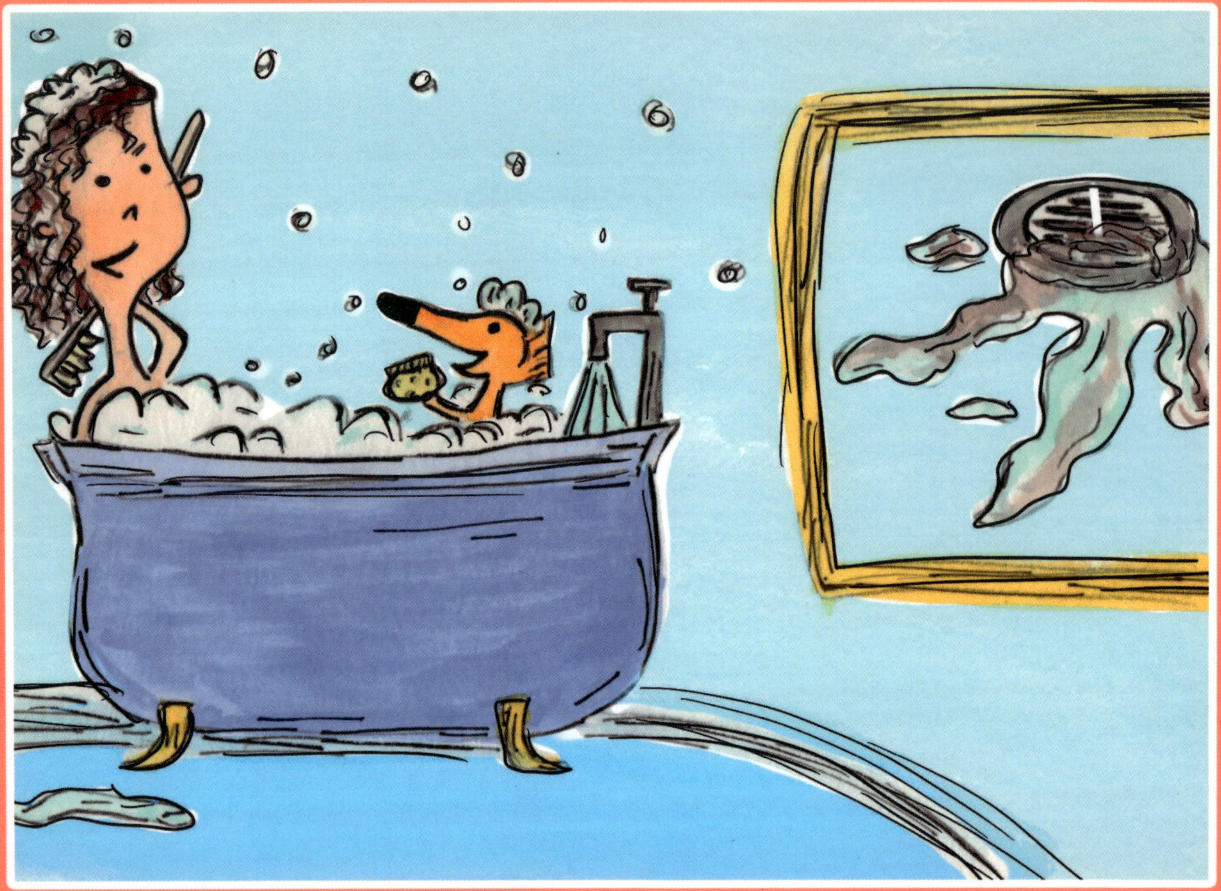

The STRENGTH of my SCARS®

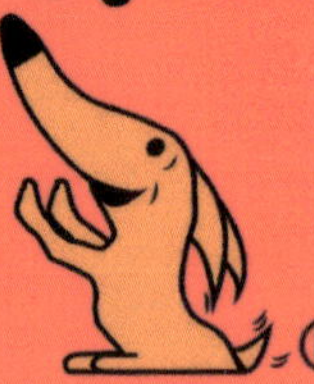

CAMBRIDGE UNIVERSITY PRESS

ISBN 978-1-00-954634-8

9 781009 546348 >

Peritoneal Dialysis:

A Bath for my Belly

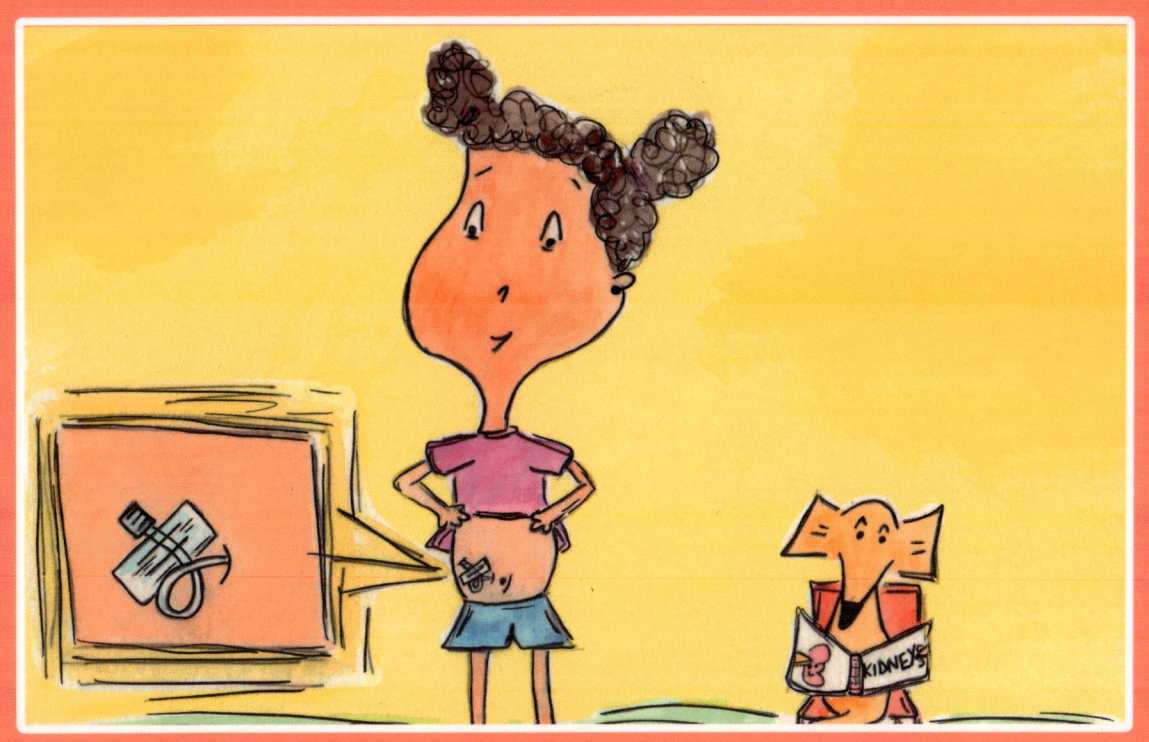

written & illustrated by Maria Baimas-George MD MPH

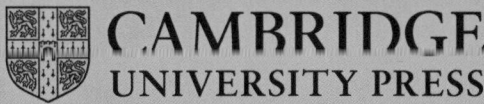

Edited by Lianna Baimas-George

Shaftesbury Road, Cambridge CB2 8EA, United Kingdom

One Liberty Plaza, 20th Floor, New York, NY 10006, USA

477 Williamstown Road, Port Melbourne, VIC 3207, Australia

314–321, 3rd Floor, Plot 3, Splendor Forum, Jasola District Centre, New Delhi – 110025, India

103 Penang Road, #05-06/07, Visioncrest Commercial, Singapore 238467

Cambridge University Press is part of Cambridge University Press & Assessment, a department of the University of Cambridge. We share the University's mission to contribute to society through the pursuit of education, learning and research at the highest international levels of excellence.

www.cambridge.org

Information on this title: www.cambridge.org/9781009546348

First published 2024

Printed in Mexico by Litográfica Ingramex, S.A. de C.V.

A catalogue record for this publication is available from the British Library.

A Cataloging-in-Publication data record for this book is available from the Library of Congress.
ISBN 978-1-009-54634-8 Paperback